HERBAL ACNE HEALING

Natural Methods to Vanish Your Acne!

Disclaimer

What Will You Find in This Book?

You open your eyes to a new day with the rays of the sun peeking through the curtains over your windows. You yawn, stretch and sleepily get out of bed. You make your way to the bathroom, bleary eyed, enter it, open the tap to let the water through, gather the water in your hands to splash it over your face, and then look at yourself in the mirror.

That's when you see it! Your heart skips a beat, and you get closer to the mirror and see that tiny little devil, rearing its ugly head and trying to make its way to the surface. Yes, you guessed it right, we are talking about none other than the pimple, those tiny little zits which try to ruin the day for you. Not only do they itch, they also distract your eyes, every time you see them on your face.

Once acne appears on your skin, it becomes very difficult to get rid of it, and even if it does disappear quickly, it leaves blemishes and dark marks, which make your skin, look dull and lifeless. So, how best to tackle this problem? Buying medicines or going to the dermatologist is very expensive and time consuming. You must be wondering whether there is any way of solving this problem at home.

Your search has finally ended, for you have come across the right book for your needs. If acne is what is troubling you and you are looking for herbal solutions, which can be prepared at home, then Herbal Acne Healing answers all of your questions. It contains a guide to various herbs and herbal solutions, which can heal acne without leaving those blemishes or dark marks.

Here is a sneak peek of what's in store for you in the book.

1. A description of what acne really is, why it occurs, and how to prevent it.
2. The different herbs and natural substances, which can be used to prevent and heal acne.
3. The process of selecting the right herb for your specific needs.
4. In addition, a 60 day plan to help you overcome your acne issues and solve them for good.

Are you ready to start learning the different remedies for acne, which are presented in this book?

Then do not waste anymore of your precious time and Start Reading Now!

Contents

What is Acne?

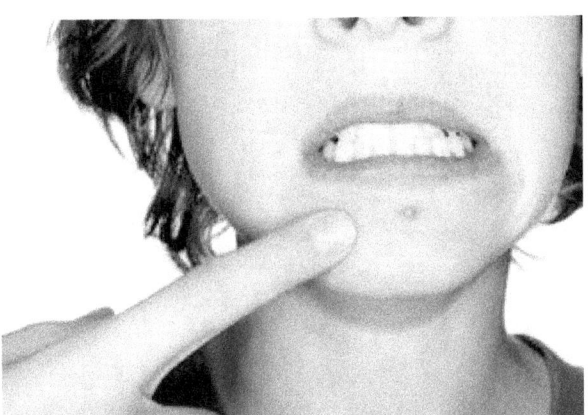

Acne Vulgaris, more commonly referred to as Acne is a skin disease, which involves the oil glands, which are located at the base of hair follicles. While acne is not dangerous to skin at all, it can result in damage such as scars and blemishes once it has occurred. Human skin consists of many pores, which are connected to the oil glands. There are many oil glands, which are present under the skin, which connect to the pores through follicles. Follicles are small canals, which transfer the oil to the pores.

The oil glands produce Sebum, which is an oily liquid. The purpose of the sebum is to carry dead skin cells, through the canals (follicles) to the skin. When the sebum reaches the surface of the skin, a small hair grows out of it, through the follicles. When the hair is not given room for growth i.e. when the follicles get blocked, the oil gets trapped and accumulates under the skin, and pimples start growing at the area, where blockage has occurred.

Causes of Acne

Simply put, there are three simple causes of acne, which are:

1. When the oil, i.e. sebum is over produced.
2. When the dead skin cells start shedding irregularly, thereby, irritating the hair follicles of your skin.
3. When bacteria starts building up on your skin.

As mentioned previously acne occurs when the follicle gets blocked, thereby, resulting in the emergence of pimples. However, due to external situations and internal conditions of the body, the problem of acne can worsen. What might these factors, which can aggregate acne, be? Let's find out.

1. **Hormones:** Many experts believe the primary factor, which causes acne, is Androgen. It is a type of hormone, which rises in its level when a human reaches adolescence. When the Androgen levels rise, they affect the oil glands, which are present under the skin, and causes them to grow further. Because of this effect, the glands start producing more oil, thereby, resulting in acne.
2. **Medications:** There are certain types of medicines, which can cause acne, like those, which contain corticosteroids, androgens, and lithium. Such drugs have been seen to cause acne in people who take them.

3. **Diet:** Improper diet can often cause acne. There are even certain dietary factors, like foods which are rich in carbohydrates, and fats, like oil, bagels, chips, etc. Along with those foods, any which have a tendency to increase the sugar level of the blood, may trigger an over production of oil from the oil glands, hence resulting in acne.

Contrary to popular opinion, foods, which are greasy, do not cause acne, nor does chocolate. It is also a common perception that dirty skin causes acne, that fact too, is incorrect.

Herbal Remedies for Acne

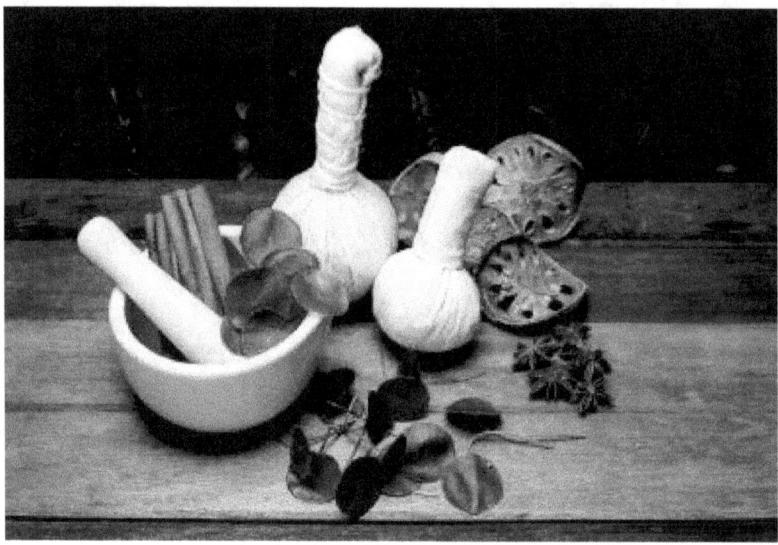

The treatment of acne through herbal means is not difficult at all. All you need to do is have the right ingredients, in the right quantities, and voila, you can whip up a solution or concoction right in the confines of your home. All of the herbal remedies mentioned in this book are directed at treating the altered pattern of acne and reducing the inflammation by producing an anti-inflammatory effect.

Following are several plant-based solutions for treating acne and ensuring that it does not occur again.

Selecting the Right Herb

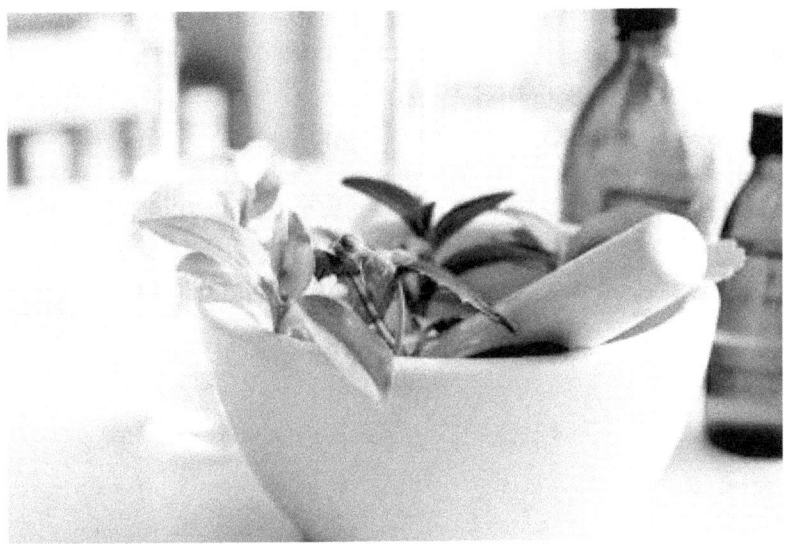

Before we tell you about the different recipes and ingredients you should use in treating your acne, you should know the difference between herbs along with when to make use of which herb.

There are different herbs, which contain properties, that not only soothe the lesions associated with acne, but also heal them. Some herbs can be used on their own, while others need to be combined with different herbs, in order to achieve the desired effect. Some types of herbs need to be applied directly to the skin, while others need to be taken so that they can ward off the acne from inside the body.

The herbs, which are popular for their lymphatic treatment properties are mostly used in herbal remedies. The combination of sarsaparilla, yellow dock, burdock herbs and cleavers is supposed to be exceptionally beneficial for warding off acne. The combination of these materials is supposed to be taken internally. You must take half a teaspoon three times a day, for it to take effect and achieve the fullest benefits.

There are other herbs as well, which must be taken to heal acne and prevent it from occurring again. Taking basil, oregano or Echinacea, will also help you in preventing acne, particularly the painful pimples that have puss in them. All three of these herbs can also be applied to the skin, which makes them even more useful. While Echinacea can be applied on the face, particularly on blemishes and the uprooted acne as is, basil and oregano, need to be applied in their oil form.

Hazelnut oil, tea tree oil, and oregano oil, are three of the most popular oils, which are used for the treatment of acne. Hazelnut oil possesses unique properties, which have the power to kill bacteria and cure acne, while tea tree oil has the ability to offer many different types of treatments. It particularly consists of anti-microbial properties, which ensures that there is an absence of bacteria wherever they are applied. Since it provides these two properties, it has the ability to reduce inflammation and gradually eliminate the outbursts of acne in the form of pimples.

Thyme essential oil is oil, which holds popularity in healing acne and acne related issues. However, do not make the mistake of applying it directly to the skin, instead add a few drops of grape seed oil in it, and then apply it, this will ensure maximum results.

Amaranth

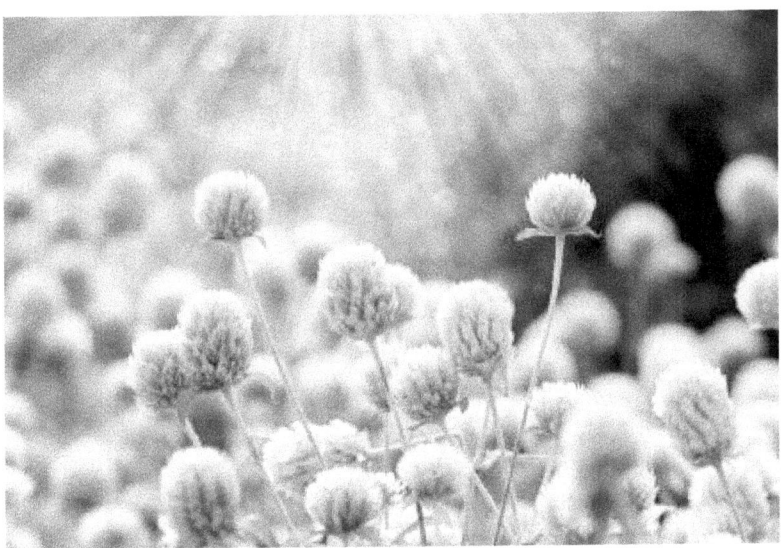

These are seeds, which are mostly found in Mexico and China. The seeds and leaves of this plant are used for treating various types of skin problems, one of which is acne. The main constituents of this herb are saponins, from which face washes may be created, and then applied on the face to reduce the inflammation of pores and heal acne.

Asparagus

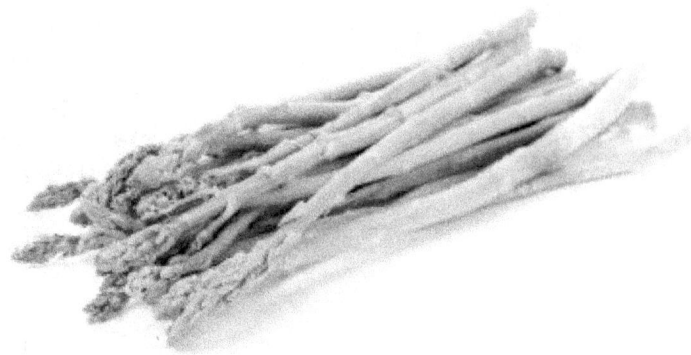

Asparagus is a perennial herb, which is mostly found in European and American regions. The fleshy roots and seeds can be used for medicinal purposes, which include treating acne. The asparagus roots consist of insulin and other materials, which can greatly reduce acne lesions and blemishes. The extract of the shoots is mostly used for cleansing the face, and has been seen to significantly improve skin appearance through acne reduction.

Jojoba oil

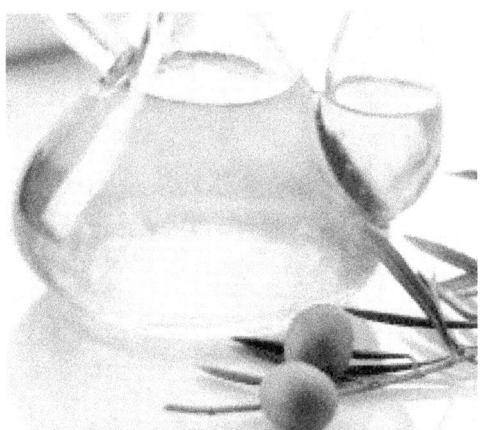

This is another great example of oil, which treats acne to the point of extinction. The oil is extracted from the jojoba seeds, and then used to cure different types of ailments, with acne being one of them. The jojoba oil is colourless and odourless, making it very easy to use and apply.

Coriander

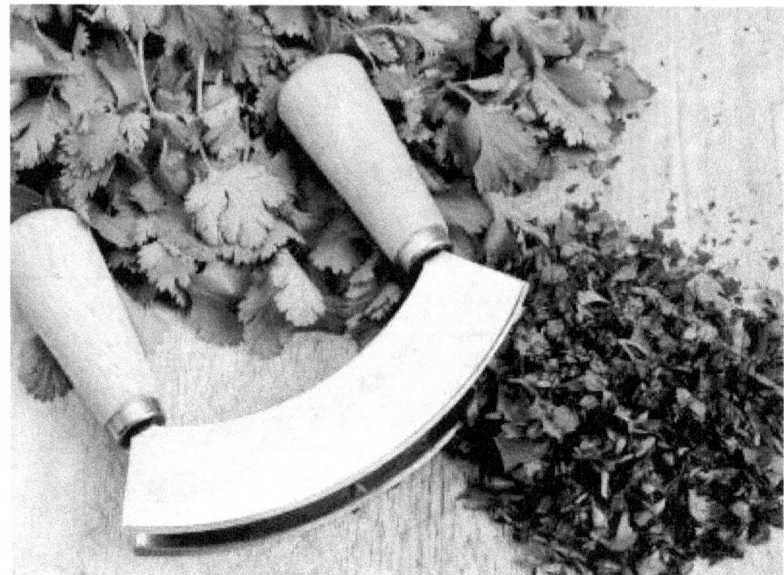

This herb is native to the Mediterranean, Asia, South Africa, Europe and America. The oil extracted from coriander is used for the treatment of acne, as it has antifungal and antibacterial properties, which makes it an excellent remedy for acne vulgaris.

Lavender Oil

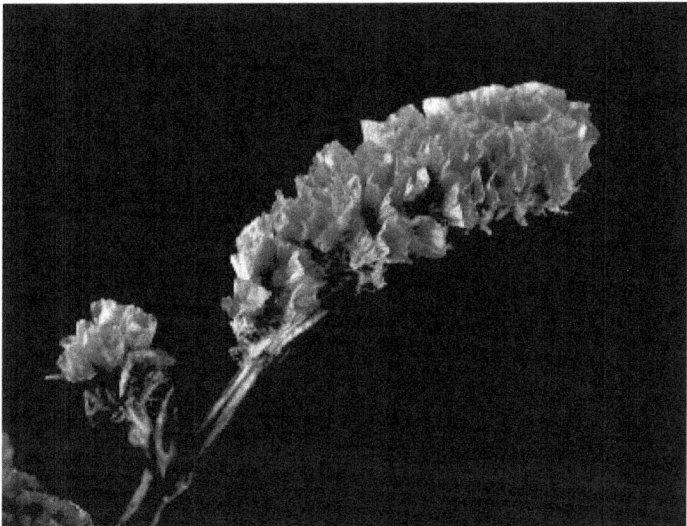

Lavender oil is another brilliant herbal remedy for the treatment of acne. The oil consists of more than 150 compounds, making it one of the most complex structured oils. Its unique composition helps to clear the skin of blemishes caused by acne, making it more radiant than ever before.

Lemon

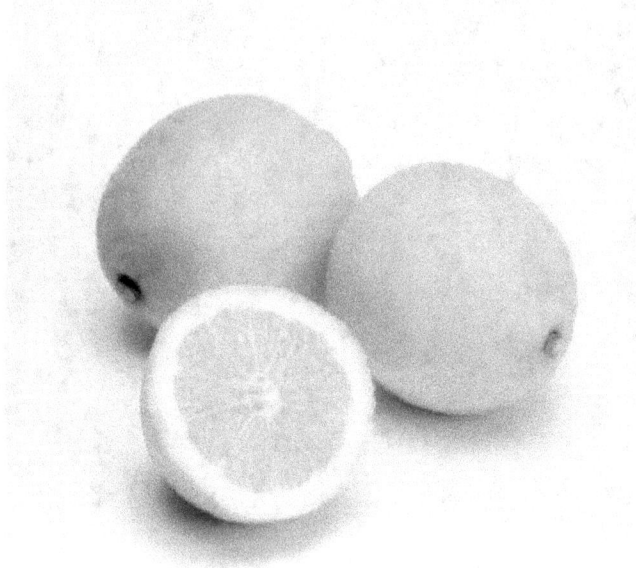

Lemon is another excellent example of an ingredient, which can not only reduce acne but also clear the dark spots on the skin, which are the result of pimples. Its antiseptic properties have the power to reduce the inflammation caused by the acne and its bleaching ability helps reduce the dark marks on the skin. This is the reason why lemon is mostly used as a bleaching agent.

Orange Peel

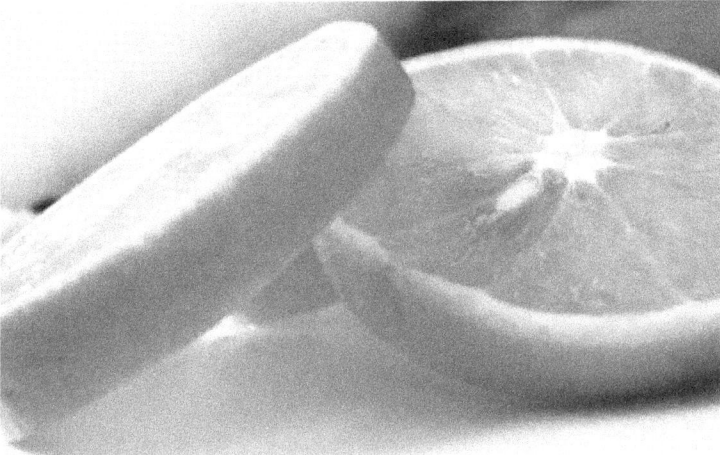

The peel of an orange is packed full of surprises. Particularly when the peel is set out to dry and pulsed to form a fine powder once dried, it can greatly help reduce the lesions caused by acne. The juice as well as the milk pastes created by mixing the dried peel with milk, is specially used for healing acne. It makes one of the best treatments of acne available.

Neem

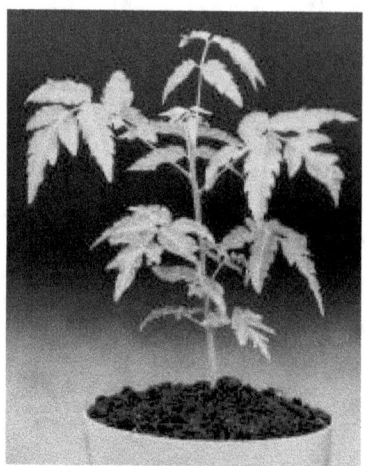

The Neem tree, whether it is the bark, leaves, branches or seeds, all exhibit medicinal properties. It can be used for the treatment of acne, by blending fresh Neem leaves with a little bit of water and pulsing until a fine puree is formed. Then apply this mixture over your face. Do not worry if it starts to itch, sometimes a lot.The antibacterial properties in Neem help in the prevention of acne and reduce the blemishes caused by it. Make sure not to let this mixture enter your eyes or mouth, for Neem is extremely bitter and you will have a highly unpleasant experience if you taste it.

Since the plant has antimicrobial properties, along with antibacterial and anti-inflammatory properties, it is one of the most effective herbal remedies for curing acne along with the dark marks caused by it.

Pine

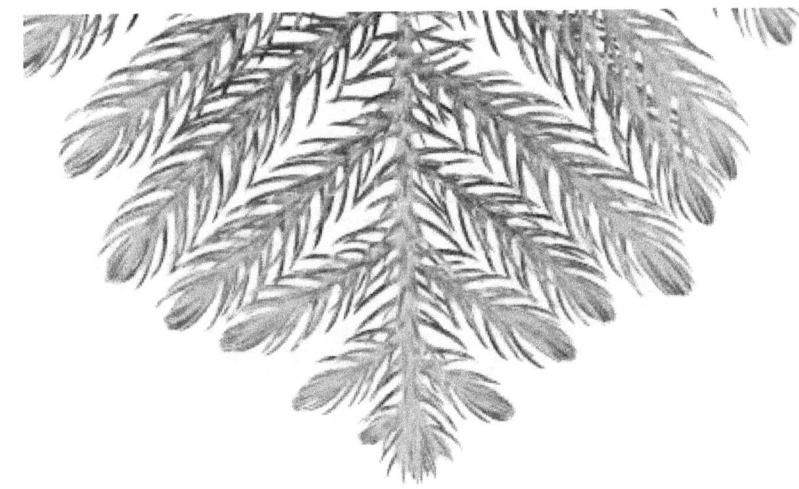

Most of the herbs are essential when it comes to treating acne from the confines of your home, none more so than pine. Pycnogenol is the main constituent of pine, which is highly recommended for the treatment of acne. Therefore, use it to ensure that your skin remains fresh and smooth, without breakouts.

Honey

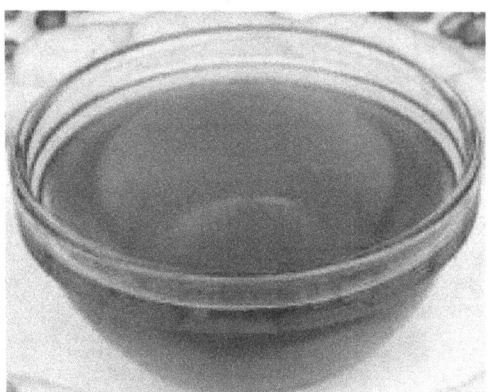

Honey is said to possess the power of healing. Experts suggest that taking honey everyday can, in fact, save you from many diseases, from the most basic, to even the most severe. Applying honey combined with powdered cinnamon, directly on the breakouts or pimples will ensure that the pimple disappears overnight without leaving a mark. Just try out this easy herbal remedy and find out for yourself.

Tea Tree Oil

As mentioned previously tea tree oil is actually very beneficial when it comes to solving acne related problems. This oil is exceptionally therapeutic in nature and is obtained by distilling the leaves through steam. This oil is extremely effective in healing acne, and ensuring that all the blemishes leave without trace.

What you need to remember about herbal remedies and healing solutions for acne is that it takes time for the applied remedy to take effect. The reason for this is that it is a completely natural healing process, and therefore, takes its time to give you the results, so do not expect them immediately. However, the best part about using herbal acne healing is that it has no side effects, which makes it all the more attractive, particularly if you are suffering from excessively painful breakouts.

Thyme

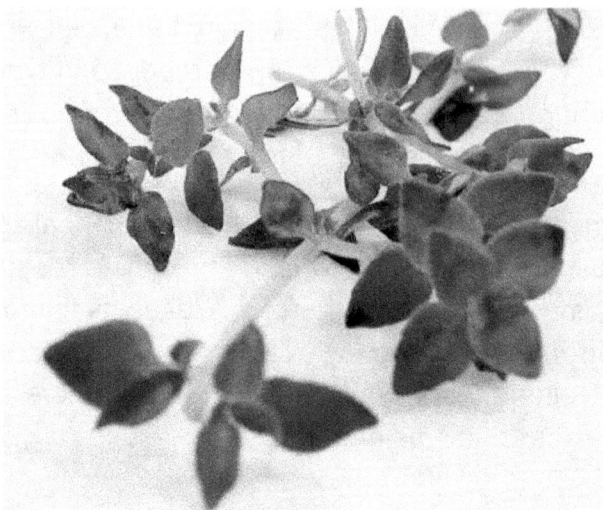

Thyme is another very important element, which is often used in the treatment of acne. The salves, prepared from the leaves of thyme, are an excellent remedy for most skin related problems, like burns, cuts, scars, and rashes. It is even more effective in curing acne and ensuring that you regain the flawless and youthful skin you possessed before these unsightly and irritating little breakouts appeared.

Mint

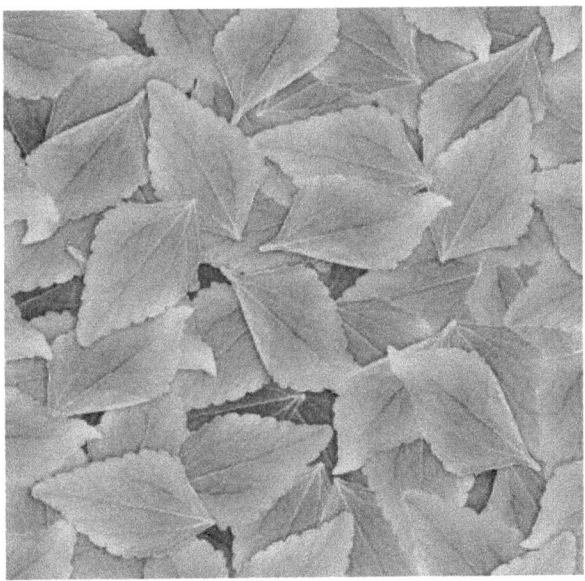

The thing about acne is that not only is it affected by external forces, rather it often occurs due to internal problems as well. Something such as acidity, which occurs as a result of anxiety, too much stress or from taking tension could cause outbreaks. Cleansing the body also helps when you want to address and cure your acne problem, once and for all. All you need to do, is take a sprig of mint, tear all the leaves from it, make sure that you have enough to fill the palms of your hands, place these leaves in a container filled with water and then let it boil until the mint and water concoction starts to turn murky brown in colour. Once you are done with this let the water boil for 4-5 minutes, and then take it off heat and set aside until it starts to cool down. Then drain the water in another container let it cool and drink it. It will help cleanse the body from all the impurities, thereby resulting in less and less breakouts every day.

Treatment of Acne – A 60 Day Plan

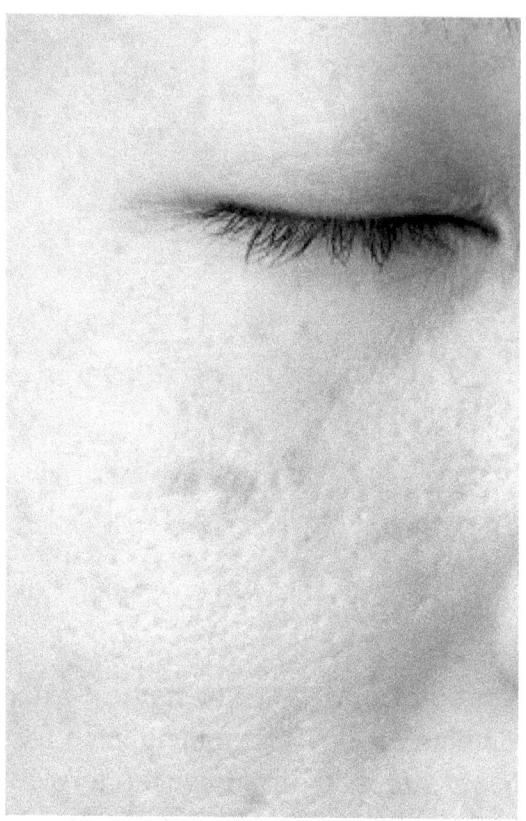

Now that you have gained an understanding of the different types of herbs, which are used for healing acne, let us explain some remedies, which can be used to make sure that the breakouts do not occur again, so that you can have radiant and beautiful skin, which is free of acne.

So, are you ready to find out the different treatments which are available in your very own home? Simple every day ingredients and yet you never knew about their secret abilities. Yes? Then let us get started on this 60-day journey of obtaining flawless skin.

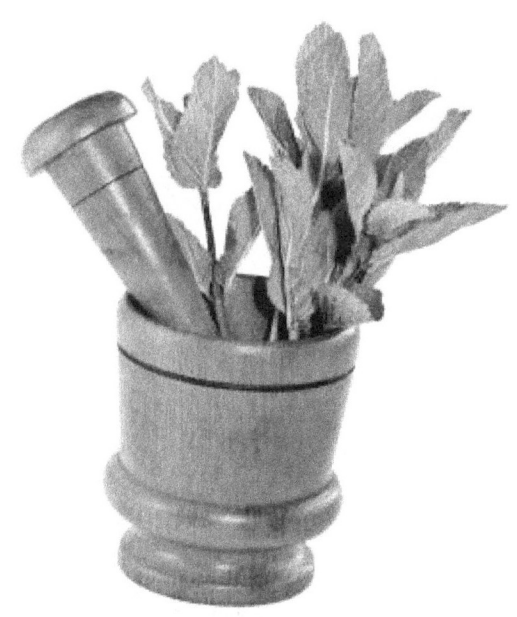

Making herbal remedies at home is extremely easy. All you need to do is locate the ingredients in your pantry, follow the instructions given in this book for making the herbal remedy, and voila, you will have an herbal solution prepared in no time at all. Following are simple herbal recipes, which can be easily prepared at home.

Turmeric and Coriander

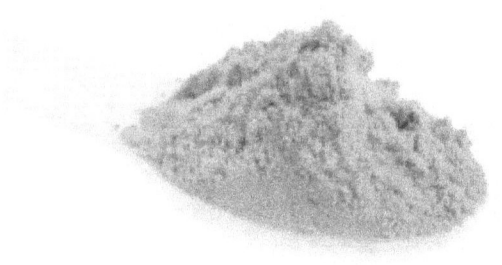 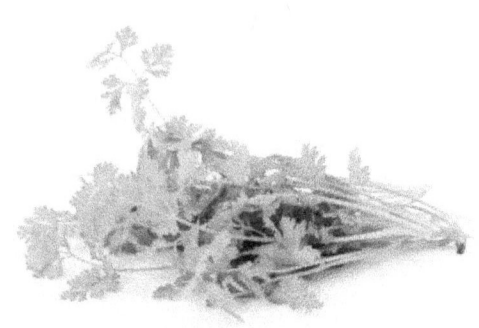

2 tsp fresh coriander juice

A pinch of turmeric

Combine the two ingredients together and mix until well incorporated. Apply daily on the entire face 2-3 times in a day. Keep this up for 7 days.

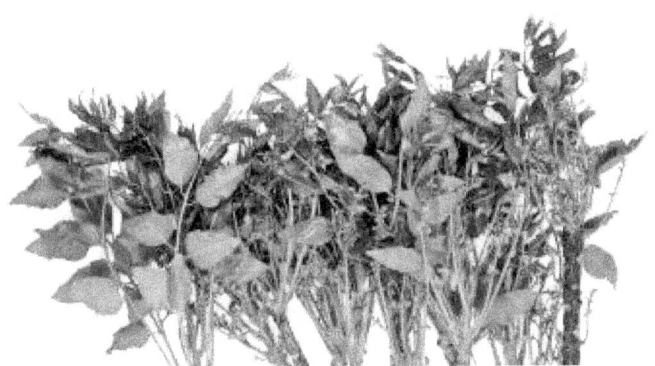

As mentioned previously, Neem whether fresh or dried is exceptionally beneficial for acne. Here are two remedies, which can be used for the treatment of acne and speed up its healing process.

Remedy 1

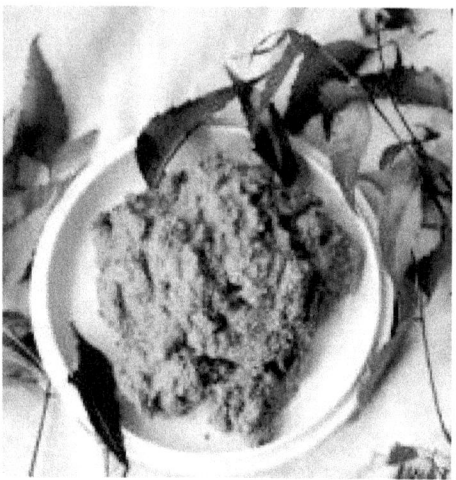

Take fresh Neem leaves, place them in a blender, and add very little water, enough for the Neem leaves to blend easily and then pulse until it forms a smooth mixture. Make sure that you have taken enough leaves, so that the resulting mixture can be applied to the entire face. Then apply this mixture, once daily, and see the results take effect right before your eyes. Follow this remedy for 60 days.

Remedy 2

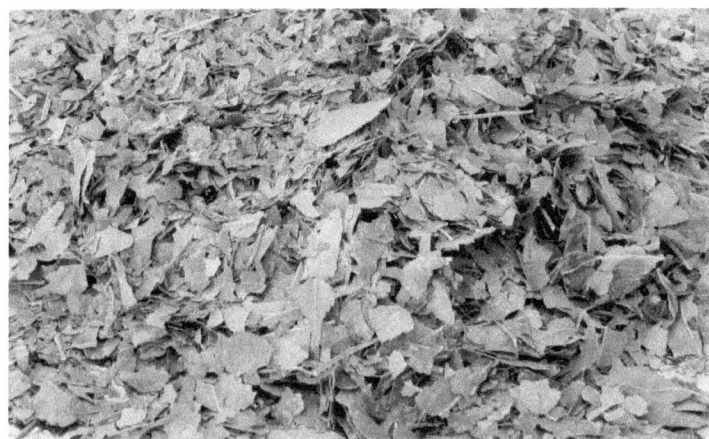

Take fresh Neem leaves dry them out by placing them in a shaded area, and then pulse until they form a powder. Once you are done, mix the dried Neem leaves with water, enough for it to take the shape of a scrub and apply once a week for 60 days, and feel the difference on your skin.

Orange Peel

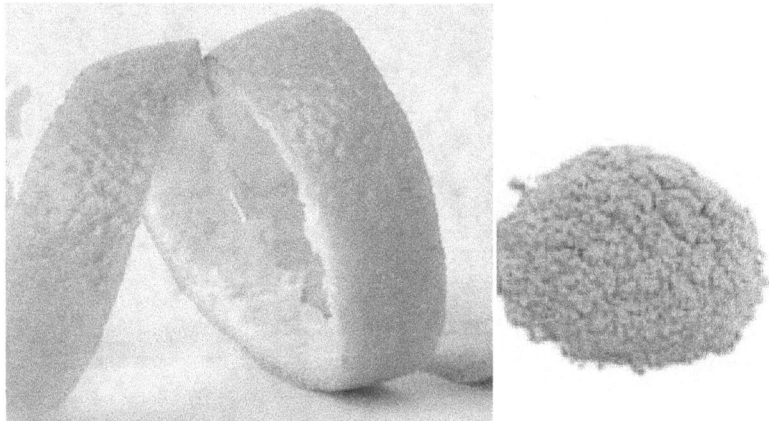

Take dried orange peels, and pulse them until they attain the form of a powder. Once you are done with this, simply mix a small amount of the orange peel powder with fresh milk, enough to make a smooth paste, apply it on your face, daily for 5-10 minutes, then rinse with cool water. Keep doing this every day for 60 days.

Rose Water

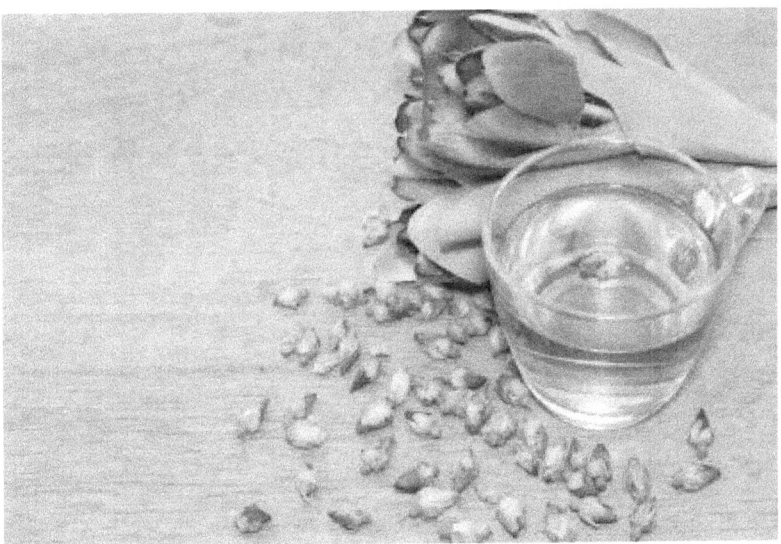

Take a fresh rose, tear the petals from it carefully, and then place a handful of them in a small saucepan filled with water. Let the water boil before adding the petals in it. Once you have placed the petals in the water, take a wooden spoon and with its help keep the rose petals in the water until they are submerged. Cover the saucepan with a lid and allow the water to cool, while letting the rose petals remain submerged in the water. Drink this water every day for cleansing your body; it will help clear out the blockages, which are resulting in the breakouts on your face.

You can also apply it on your face for a healthy glow. Either apply it as a wet pack or simply wash your face 2-3 times in a day with this freshly created rose water.

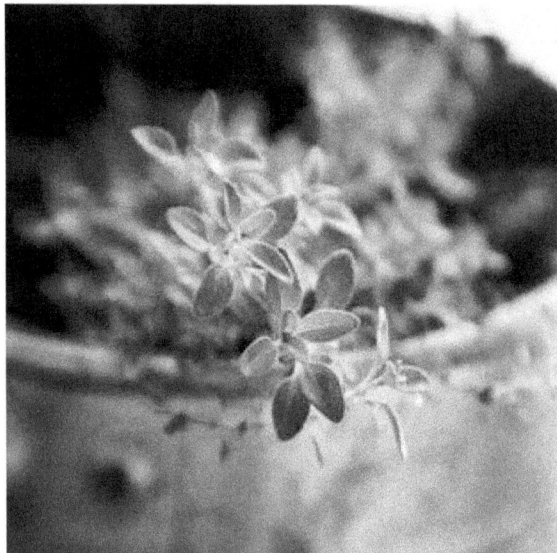

We have already discussed how thyme salve is used for the treatment of acne; it speeds up the healing process and helps in removing traces of acne from the skin. You can make a thyme salve at home as well, all you need are the right ingredients, in the right amounts and you will have everything you need to get started.

Take pure ghee, place it in a saucepan and allow it to warm, enough for it to start bubbling without burning. Add in two handfuls of coarsely chopped fresh thyme leaves in this heated ghee, and then lower the heat to very slow, cover the saucepan with a lid and then let it simmer and cook gently for an hour. Then strain the mixture through a coarse wire sieve and place the drained mixture into the saucepan once again, placing it back on heat. Cover it again and let it heat up for 5 minutes. Remove the lid after that and add in two tablespoons of bees wax and ½ teaspoon of pure vanilla, stirring it all the while until the bees wax is thoroughly combined.

Now it is done, pour the mixture out into jars, making sure that the jars are not too deep. Let the mixture set, only after that, secure the top of the jars with a lid. Keep them in a dry and cool place. Take a small portion of this mixture every day and apply it on your face, massaging it lightly over the entire area. Repeat this process everyday once you have created the mixture and then apply it once after taking a bath and at night before sleeping. Experience the thyme salve take effect in front of your very eyes.

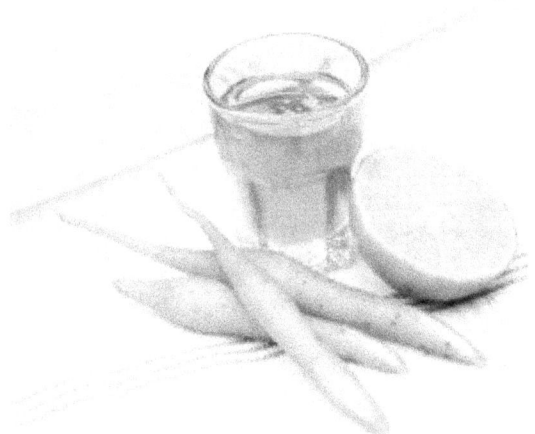

Mixing lemon and honey will help you get rid of pimples, as well as the dark marks, which come with them. Simply slice the lemon in half, add one or two drops of honey over it, and then squeeze the lemon lightly to mix the honey, then apply the lemon on your face, while squeezing the lemon. This will apply the lemon juice mixed with honey on your face. The honey will help get rid of the pointy heads of acne, while the lemon will help in getting rid of the marks. This is an exceptionally helpful remedy, which works well on all types of skin, particularly for oily skin.

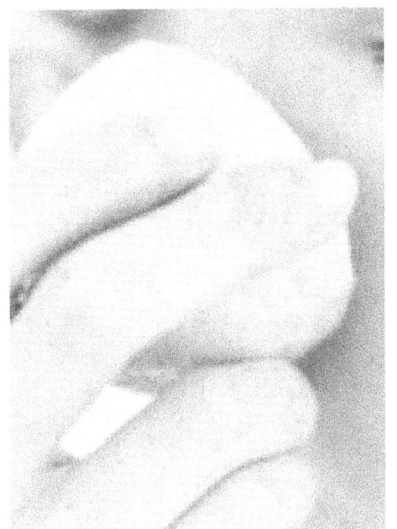

Aloe Vera

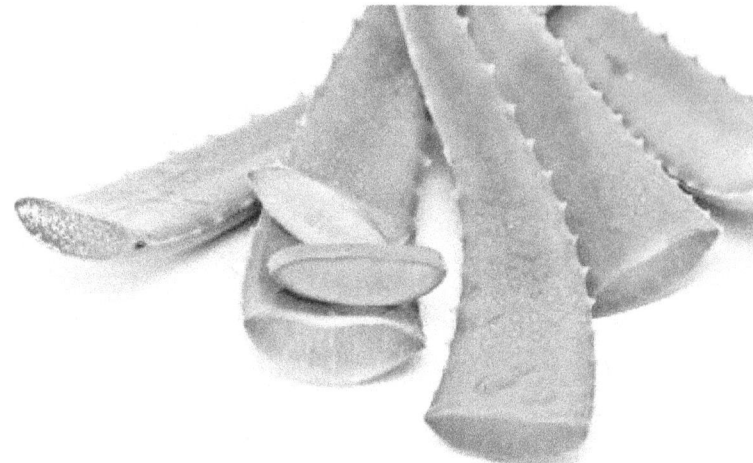

Apply the freshly squeezed pulp of Aloe Vera on your face, and see the acne disappear.

Honey and Cinnamon

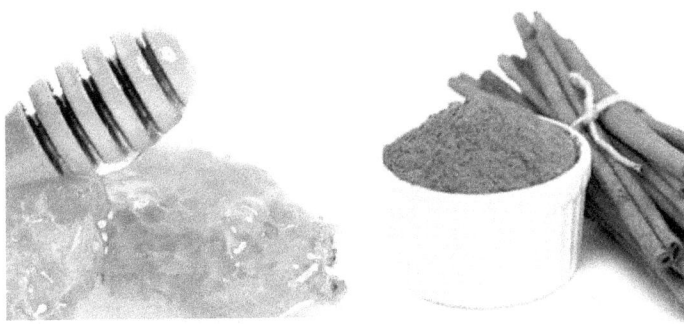

Mix a tablespoon of honey with a pinch of cinnamon powder, stir until well combined and then dip your finger in it, and dab your pimple with this mixture. This remedy works exceptionally well when you only have a couple of pimples on your face and not a severe case of acne. Every time a pimple pops up use this remedy.

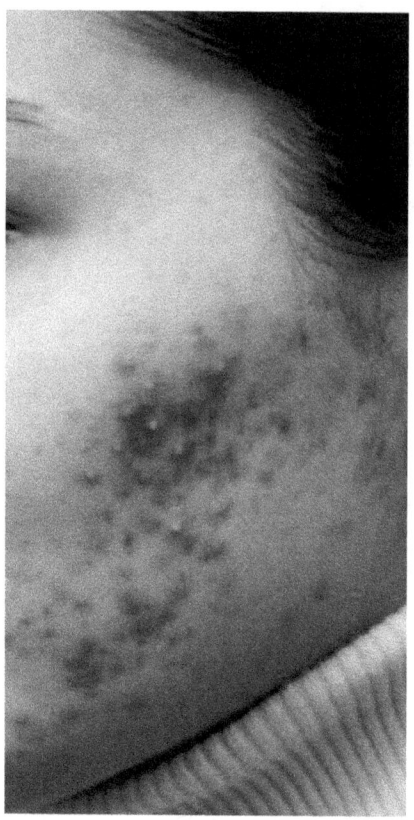

In the previous section, you learned about the different types of remedies, which can be made at home, and applied to the acne affected areas. In this section we mentioned a simple acne healing plan for 60 days, after following it, your skin will not only be clear of acne and its marks, but it will glow and shine, like healthy skin does.

This 60 day plan is very simple, all you have to do is apply the remedies mentioned in the previous section in the following order.

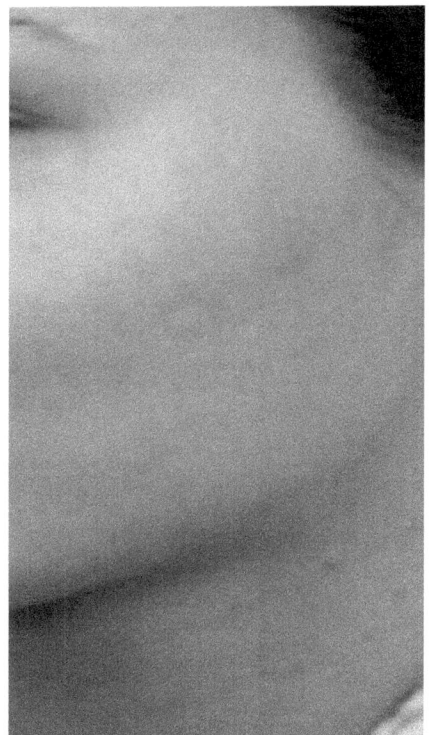

Wake up fresh in the morning and apply the orange powder mixed with water or fresh milk on your face. Leave it for 15 minutes. Then wash your face with cool water. Do not rub the skin when you apply the paste; it will wash off easily when you apply water over it.

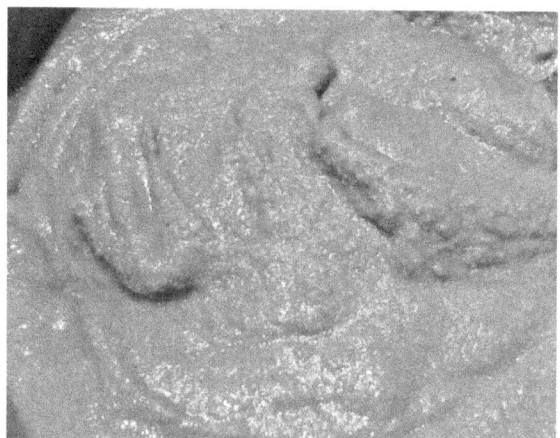

After washing your face, apply the coriander and turmeric mixture. Leave it on for 5 – 10 minutes, then rinse with cool water.

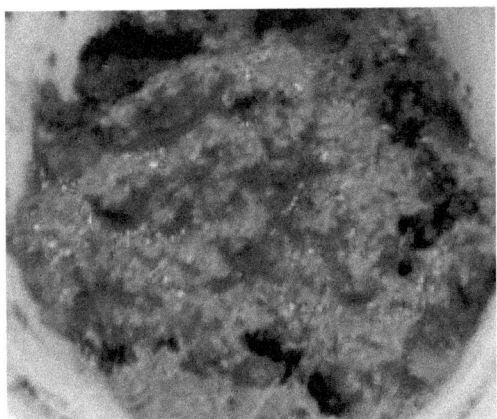

Apply the Neem paste on your face after you have had your lunch, make sure not to let the mixture go into your eyes or mouth, it is extremely sour. If it goes in your eyes, simply rinse them with water a couple of times. When you are applying this paste, make sure not to rub too harshly; in fact in the initial stages simply apply it without massaging. It will itch a lot, as the Neem will act against the acne and cure it, so you will have to bear with it. Leave it for 15 minutes, then rinse with cold water.

Apply rose water afterwards.

Evening

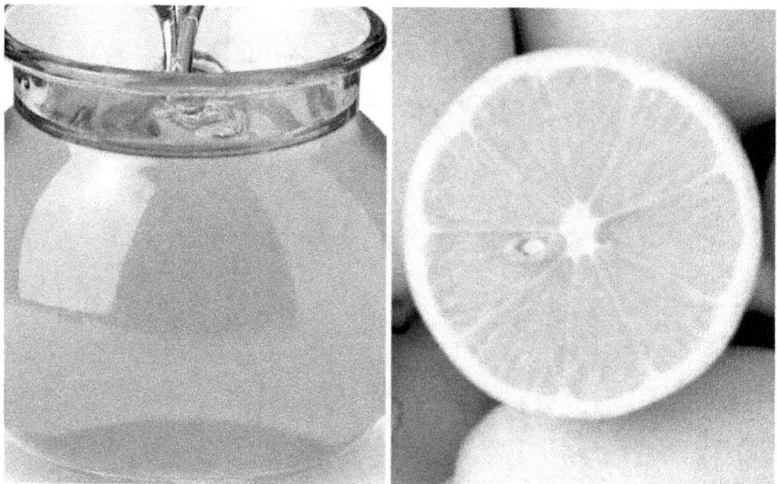

Apply the lemon and honey mixture on your face, the lemon with sting a little, as it works to cure your acne. Be patient with the itchiness you feel. Leave it on for 15 to 20 minutes, then rinse with water, while massaging gently. Make sure that the lemon and honey mixture is completely rinsed off.

NOTE: Do not go out in the sun after applying the lemon and honey mixture, the sun rays will react with the lemon and tan your skin.

After you are done with this, have a glass of rose water.

Night

Before you sleep, apply the thyme salve, after preparing it by following the instructions given above. Leave it on for a couple of minutes, before rinsing with cold rose water.

Make sure not to rub too aggressively in the initial three weeks. You will see the acne clearing as the weeks' progress. When you start this herbal healing process, make sure to drink lots of water throughout the day. Also, drink rose water at least once every day. After three weeks, start massaging your face gently, following the same process for the entire day, i.e. morning through night. Keep following this herbal remedy for 60 days and embrace the radiant and beautiful acne free skin you have.

Make sure to follow the process as mentioned above and do not try to pair any herbal remedy with the other, for it might result in unwanted consequences. If you want to make any changes, make sure to consult an herbal treatment expert, otherwise follow this healing plan, and gain the benefits it offers.

Obtaining Acne Free Skin

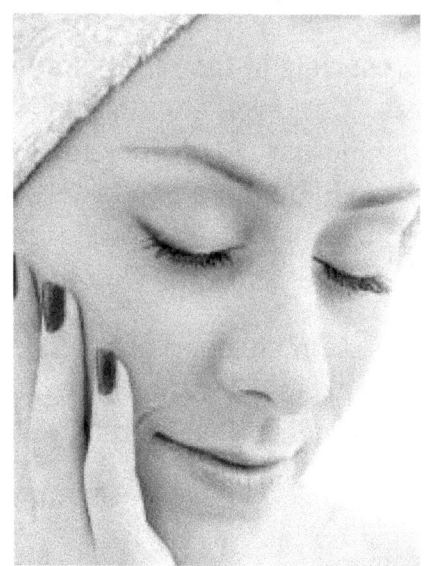

Obtaining acne free skin is not something, which will happen with magic. Sure, you can take medicines for it, but then keep in mind that medicines come with their own share of side effects as well. Herbal healing procedures and treatment options are not only healthy for you but also are free from side effects or reactions.

Obtaining skin, which is healthy, radiant, and free from acne, is easy once you are aware of the different types of herbal treatments available, and those, which take you hardly any time to whip up. Apply them on your face, as instructed and feel the difference they make to your skin, after a couple of days. One thing, which must be remembered in acne healing, is that it takes time, so you have to be patient and wait for the results. The results will not appear overnight and your scars will not vanish in just a day or two. You will have to work hard and keep at it for a couple of months to get the desired result, which is a healthy and flawless skin complexion, completely free of acne.

So what are you waiting for?

Start following the herbal remedies provided in the book, and become one step closer to obtaining the beautiful skin which is hiding beneath your acne and its scars.

End Note

Peruse the pages of the book, and find out all you need to know about herbal acne healing, the different types of herbal remedies, which can be prepared at home and how they can be beneficial for your skin. Herbal remedies offer you an exceptionally effective way of dealing with your acne problem.

The healing process, while it takes a lot of time, it is so effective, that even once you are free from acne, you would want to continue it. Herbal treatments for acne have many benefits; the biggest benefit is that it is a completely natural method of curing acne. So make sure to utilize this method when you want to deal with all of your acne or related problems.

This book provides everything you need to know about herbal acne healing, so go through the pages and get enlightened regarding the different remedial recipes, and curing solutions, which will make this acne nightmare seem like a thing of the past.